REBECCA FINE

Mind Your Mouth

Improving your relationship with food one bite at a time

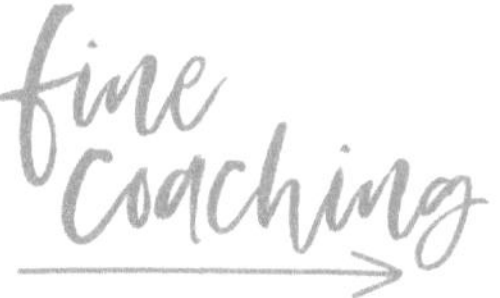

Contents

Chapter One   1
  What is Mindful or Intuitive Eating?   1
Chapter Two   9
  Why Is Mindful Eating So Important?   9
Chapter Three   17
  Preparing For Mindful Eating   17
Chapter Four   25
  Putting Mindful Eating into Practice   25
Chapter Five   30
  Tips for Mindful Eating   30
Chapter Six   37
  The Benefits of Eating With Family and Friends   37
  The Challenges of Eating with Others   40
Chapter Seven   45
  Commonly Asked Questions   45

1

Chapter One

What is Mindful or Intuitive Eating?

Mindful eating is a very powerful concept that can alter your life in profound ways.

Rooted in ancient Buddhist teachings, mindful eating aims to connect us deeply to the pleasure of eating, helping us foster a healthy relationship with food, curb cravings, eliminate binge eating and heighten our awareness of the variety and quality of the meals we consume. When practiced daily, mindful eating, or intuitive eating as is it also known, is quite the opposite of a typical 'weight loss' diet, being hinged on the concept that there is no right or wrong way to eat, but rather varying degrees of consciousness about what we are eating and why. It's not hard to imagine the number of people who struggle with lifestyle diseases such as obesity, diabetes, eating disorders, high blood pressure and heart disease, not to mention those with depression, anxiety, ADHD, even a general lack of self worth. In todays fast paced society we tend to be focused on what and how much as opposed to when and why. There are hundreds of millions of people across the world that could draw immense benefits from bolstering their resolve around food with mindful eating.

You are probably wondering, if this is such a powerful concept, that's been around for so long..then why aren't people practicing it already? Well, the truth is that many people in modern society are not fully aware of what mindful eating is. It's typically not something we grew up with, so kudos to you for picking up this book. You are going to learn just how easy and effective mindful eating can be and how beautifully its benefits weave themselves through the entire tapestry of your life, even with a busy schedule, a hectic family life or limited meal choices.

Let's start by defining what mindful eating is

Mindful eating is closely related to the more widely comprehended concept of "Mindfulness". Defined as 'a mental state achieved by focusing one's awareness on the present moment, while calmly acknowledging and accepting one's feelings, thoughts, and bodily sensations.', mindfulness is a concept that is congruent with a growing number of professionals and individuals alike who are awakening to the benefits of active, intentional consciousness in life's pursuits. In whatever you are doing, by being mindful you are simply putting your mind and all your senses into your current activity. This enables you to be present with your whole being and to be aware of everything in your environment and emotions not just the mechanics of the task at hand.

Mindful eating, therefore, refers to bringing your whole self to your dinner table. It means concentrating your heart, soul and all five senses to the flavors and textures of your food, the locations where you take meals, the company you dine with, and the emotions associated with those foods as you chew. This includes snacks you may take in between meals. Observing your rituals around food in this manner becomes akin to a personal super power, helping you discover more about your general eating habits, especially those triggers that spur less desirable consumption preferences and even your mood during meals. Also, as your practice deepens, you may find your notions of what you choose to eat shifting dramatically for the better too. This gives you a simple yet powerful way to alter your conscious decision making right at the mouth that will carry through in many other areas of your life.

Principles of Mindful Eating

To understand mindful eating it is important that we consider the principles that guide the practice. The main principles of mindful eating are as follows:

Awareness

Mindful eating requires that you deliberately pay attention to every detail when consuming food. The taste, the smell, the texture, the colors and appearance of the food you eat are all brought to your attention with purpose. This helps you develop a better relationship with the kind of dishes you choose and why. Though such is a obvious place to start, you also need to be keenly aware of your environment. The food you eat is not independent of your environment. Think about the stark differences not only in food, but in the pace and your state of mind while eating between a drive-thru and a sit-down restaurant, typically we are scarfing down food in the former while languishing more casually in the latter. You must take notice of the environment in which the food was served, the disposition of the person who made it or served it to you, the presentation of the meal, the utensils, the materials of the table and chair you are seated at and even the quality of the air and the energy in the room.

You should also be aware of your internal environment. Eating food has a way of bringing hidden emotions to the fore of our minds. This may include pleasant emotions from the last time you tasted a similar meal, perhaps a reminder of the first time you ate it, or the people and place which hold a strong memory associated with the food. In some cases it may evoke sad or more trying emotions. Being aware of these emotions and accepting them without judgment is an important part of mindful eating. This is designed to make sure that you are not just building a healthy relationship with food but supporting yourself in becoming more self-aware, recognizing the choices you make and your accompanying thought processes. This awareness goes a long way in helping us become a better version of ourselves.

Eating Slowly

Most of us are conditioned to gulp down our food without giving any thought to its taste, texture or flavors. Often this habit leads to overeating and is the genesis of many lifestyle diseases. Mindful eating proposes the opposite of this form of mindless eating. It encourages us to eat slowly as we feel the texture, taste, and flavors and savor the experience of eating.

Eating slowly doesn't have to be an arduous extreme, but a little less haste helps you chew more of your food and this goes a long way in promoting optimal digestion. In addition, indulging in each bite, you'll discover more enjoyment of food as you give your mouth more time to feel the taste, textures and flavors in your meals. Moderating the momentum of meals also helps you become aware of the quantity of food you are eating. You'll find you get much more notice when you are close to being full and thus avoid overeating.

Hitting the brakes while eating can feel like an uphill task with kids but it is something you can achieve. By emulating the practice at the table and reminding yourself, and your family, that eating is not a race, you can instill the habit early with your little people and create the foundations of pleasurable time to connect in the long-term. You can even make a game of it with kids by seeing who can chew their food the longest or perhaps introducing chopsticks if you don't mind the extra clean up! Maybe start by putting the spoon or fork down in between bites. You should also chew your food slowly, a minimum of 20 chews is often recommended, as you feel each morsel and enjoy the many complex flavors. You will find that your mouthful becomes almost liquid at this point, an incredible benefit to your digestive system. You should also practice to take a deep breath in between bites. This will decelerate your eating considerably and allow you to take pleasure in your food even more. With flavors lingering that much longer you may start to develop a preference for higher quality, less processed foods, refining your palate naturally to a healthier variety.

Savor the Food

Savor your food simply means to choose the food that you eat. Many people don't take time to choose food that they love or those that will nourish their bodies the most. Instead, they eat food just because it is available, fast, is easy to prepare or because someone else is having the same dish. Not taking the time to care for your self by providing it with the best nutrients available for your needs does a real disservice to your body. Often, we are guilty of putting premium gas in our car and regular in our own tanks, eating purely to quench a hunger pang, to follow a habitual routine or, as in many cases, to numb unpleasant emotions. This is not how you were designed to live! Eating quickly because you sense a hunger pang generally leads to mindlessly swallowing your food, overeating and consuming without care as to how that food will help your body.

Hunger should never be the driver in meal selection as it often goes for the first thing you can put in your mouth! Instead use hunger as a cue for when to start eating and it's passing for when to stop. Hunger is one of the three parts to eating, the others being pleasure and nourishment. You have a sense of taste for a reason. To enjoy and vary what you eat. Most of us are very lucky to live in parts of the world where a wide variety of nutrients are readily available. Don't waste this precious gift on shoveling in 'franken-foods' as fast as you can! Besides, the food you choose should meet all the needs of your body, providing all the important nutrients you need to thrive.

Gratitude

A thankful heart is the beginning of all great experiences in life. Start appreciating your food even if you feel that you could have had something better. Before you take your meal, take a minute or two just to be thankful for all that you have including the food before you. Silently expressing your gratitude for the fact that you have food to eat will open your heart and soul to feel and enjoy the food when you start eating. This way you will find yourself focused on the food you are eating and feeling every flavor in it. This makes the whole experience of mindful eating natural, worthwhile and a beautiful practice to extend throughout your existence.

Take Small Portions

Often we want to take a bite to fill our entire mouth for it to count. Aside from increasing your choking risk, we've all seen someone take a bite so big they've almost had to hold it in with one hand while they chew. Hence the phrase, 'biting off more than you can chew'. In fact, mindful eating requires that you consume your food in *small bites*. Most likely, much smaller than you currently do. This leaves room in your mouth for you to chew the food thoroughly without any urge to swallow quickly. In addition, this creates room for your food to mix well with saliva so that you can pass the bite from one side of the tongue to the other, experiencing all the flavors before swallowing with ease. Many small bites grant clearer recognition of fullness, allowing you to stop before you overeat.

Be Aware of your Hunger Levels

In most schools and workplaces, lunch break is always at the same time every day. Have you noticed what happens during lunch? Everyone rushes to the canteen, café, or restaurant whether they are hungry or not. This is the time to eat, so, we eat. This is more interesting in the workplace because even employees who arrived late, having already had a morning meal and most probably not feeling hungry, will rush to have their lunch just like everyone else. You can probably see why the practice of eating at certain times rather than from the cue to eat can lead to overeating at all meals throughout the day. Intuitive eating turns this mindless routine on its head.

Mindful eating gives you the grace to eat when you are hungry and to stop eating as soon as your hunger ends. What this means is that you don't have to follow the physical clock instead you should focus on your body. It will tell you when it needs to recharge and when it is full. You are not a robot! As a living, breathing human, it is in your best interest to obey your body and not just some senseless routine. To this end, you will need to start planning your days in such a way that you only eat when you are hungry and keenly focus on your intake while eating so that you can stop at the appropriate signal. Plus, you can also use lunch to let down a little, destress, catch up socially and relish the other pleasures of a short break alone or with company. Eating optional!

2

Chapter Two

Why Is Mindful Eating So Important?

Most likely are reading this book because you want to reap the benefits of mindful eating. If this is the case, then congratulations for you are in the right place. This book has been written specifically to help you harness the powers of mindful eating to improve your life one bite at a time. However, if on the other hand, you are reading this book because perhaps are skeptical as to the effectiveness of intuitive eating, then read on! It's not just been a practice of Buddhists for thousands of years, the many health benefits both physically and mentally, have been scientifically proven. Here are just some of the benefits you will derive from including this ritual in your life:

Establishing your Ideal Weight Naturally

One of the most studied aspects of mindful eating is how, if at all, it can contribute to weight reduction. The majority of the reported studies have found that mindful eating does clearly support overweight individuals in successfully releasing weight and keeping it off. These studies really only serve to place a stamp on what millions of mindful eating practitioners have known for decades. Mindful eating augments three important criteria to releasing weight:

1. It helps cut down on consumption of unhealthy foods
2. It helps to eliminate mindless overeating
3. It helps you become the Captain of your eating habits

Mindful eating requires sharpened senses surrounding the foods you consume. This heightened awareness will begin to influence not only your food choices but the emotions that motivate those decisions in the first place. Over time, you will deliberately make healthier more varied selections regarding your daily subsistence. More preference for nutrient dense foods will result in a natural shedding of nutritionally empty foods and give your body a real chance of releasing some extra weight. Another term for this is 'crowding out' the foods you are looking to eliminate with those you wish to add.

Deliberately unhurried mealtimes, with each bite spending longer in the mouth, commonly leads to smaller portions than you would have typically eaten before you began the practice. With considerably more notice when hunger is quenched, intu-itive eating often eliminates overeating completely and hence gives you the ability to comfortably stop at the appropriate time and ultimately reset your body to it's ideal weight.

Lastly, when you start mindful eating you will learn to manage your eating habits with greater acuity. Most people with obesity remark they have no control where food is concerned. They struggle with their intake and often reach for the fatty, salty and sugary appeal of fast foods. Eating at any time food is available is also common with overeating, the combination of these two dietetic no-no's can very dangerous. One of the tools you'll acquire with mindful eating, is the mind mastery necessary to avoid impulse eating, instead following your bodies signals on when to eat, what to eat and when to stop eating. Mindful eating, even without any initial change in diet, will go a long way to honing in on this recognition of the proper signals of the body.

Aiding Digestion

Many of us suffer from indigestion and other digestive ailments simply because we are often in so much of a hurry to finish our meals that we don't give the digestive system the right time, the right food or the right conditions for smooth assimilation. This results in most of what we consume exiting the system without being entirely metabolized. By consuming food this way we miss out on many nutrients that pass through our bodies before any benefits are fully absorbed, regardless of whether the meal was considered healthy or otherwise.

Take, for example, you've had a long morning meeting and barely had time to make it to lunch. As you head out to the cafeteria you are reminded of another important meeting that is starting in the next ten minutes or so.

What would you typically do in this situation? You'd rather eat than go hungry..

Like most people we tend to quickly order the first thing on the menu, then gulp it down without even pausing to think about what those big chunks will do once they are locked inside our bodies.

The result?

Well, as there are no teeth beyond the mouth, you'll most likely begin to experience stomach unrest within several minutes. Why? Those large bites are still the same size! Now, however, they are sitting in the digestive highway causing a traffic jam and your stomach responds to this 'Mealtime 911' by producing more acid than normal to clear it away. However, this actually doesn't help you either because all this extra effort from your body now means you can't focus on the next meeting anyway. Your stomach is roiling, working overtime to 'move' things along and you can barely remain alert. Sound familiar?

The digestive system in the human body is designed to work at optimal levels when properly maintained. Overloading it can break it down. Usually, when you eat, your stomach can determine the kind of food you ingested. It's then able to tell the glands to tailor the enzyme production in order to digest that particular morsel. However, for the food to be adequately digested, it must have been chewed into such minute masses that it allows for these chemicals to flow freely between particles. When you fail to chew your food thoroughly then the enzymes cannot do their job. Meaning, a lot of helpful nutrients escape your body without being adequately soaked up. Speaking of escape, coupled with the potential to cause long term harm to your intestines, undigested food can lead to some pretty nasty smelling gas which could possibly cause harm to your social life too..

Reduce Stress and Anxiety

It has been found that many obese individuals gain weight as a result of emotional eating. It's common in those who turn to food when they encounter unpleasant emotions to reach for the more desirable experience of eating as a way to numb those difficult feelings. The truth is that food is a very powerful element in our life. Not only does it nourish our bodies and bring us together as human beings but has a huge impact on our emotions. Many people carrying excess weight dull emotions with food because of it's intense power to lull negative feelings and often distract enough to at least temporarily forget. Sadly, the long term effects of overeating are not so temporary and often those negative feelings come back double with a side helping of shame and guilt. Conversely, with the intuitive eating methods you are learning in this book, you can also use the process of consuming food to deal with your emotions, only in this case you'll also be reducing stress and anxiety in a way that will create a positive impact on your life.

We've well established that practicing mindful eating encourages you to reduce the pace of your meals. This leisurely amble with food has a way of supporting you in your emotional awareness. It's truly a form of full body meditation. As you learn to focus on your feelings as you eat, you will notice a heightened awareness of your emotional state and with deep breathing and concentration, you will concurrently develop a tool to help you deal with the more challenging emotions in your life. As you eat, hidden sentiments are likely to rush to the fore during the chewing process. Often those emotions are associated with certain foods, places, people or historical circumstances relating to that food. Learning to experience these emotions and then manage them as they come can help you reduce stress and get a grasp on anxiety.

Besides, mindful eating has a way of calming you down. Unhurried meals, with a fixation on each mouthful, leads, in essence, to a shut down of the emotions tied to other issues in the bustle of your day and for that moment, you singularly experience the pure joy of consuming food. This quiets the mind, funneling your thoughts and feelings introspectively, thus helping create a more serene mental landscape for any of life's more trying decisions. Mindful eating promotes greater emotional intelligence for weathering the challenges of change and managing stress with greater composure.

Millions of people worldwide experience a legitimate emotional grapple when they choose food as a momentary therapy for rough days, emotionally difficult situations, procrastination and even stress or avoidance at work. If you find yourself craving your favorite snack every time you encounter unpleasant situations, be it work-related stress, financial problems or even a rush of emotions from a recollection of the past, acknowledge that you may be using food to self-medicate. Eating solely to self-soothe is the largest contributor to obesity cases in the world and is a factor in many other lifestyle diseases such as high blood pressure, diabetes and even heart disease. If this is you, or someone you care about, then mindful eating offers an excellent option you can begin right now, that won't interfere with your life, doctors orders or your current palate and can immediately ease you on your way to managing a love-hate relationship with food comfortably and effectively. Practicing these methods will clarify to you why you feel the urges to eat when you aren't hungry, you'll become aware of your motivators or triggers to eat and this is the starting point for modifying your eating habits. In fact, any habit in general can be approached in this way.

Know that the awareness that comes with mindful eating can go a long way in underpinning any medical efforts to change your problematic eating habits, however, if you are struggling with chronic eating disorders please seek professional help

Developing Focus

When you practice mindful eating, you are also disciplining the rare skill of zoning in on one thing. You learn to set aside distractions and apply pinpoint concentration. The truth is, that to succeed at most *anything* in life you must know how to focus. By choosing to practice mindful eating you start to unilaterally habituate laser concentration which puts you on the path to success in other areas of your life as you develop the ability to easily close out distractions. You'll naturally repeat this exercise multiple times throughout your day as most of us eat more than once! It's no wonder apply this technique (or not) can impact so many areas of life!

Improving Your Overall Health

Ancillary improvement throughout your general health it a matter-of-course with a committed practice of intuitive eating. It's akin to *falling in love* with your food, and not the smothering

kind of obsessive love you see in scary movies, but by spotlight-
ing single-mindedness every time you have a meal or a snack,
you craft a respectful, healthy sort of love. One you will continue
to treasure. It's recognizing how the very act of eating well
positively affects all areas of your life both in your physical and
emotional nourishment. As human beings we rely on food to live
and the way in which we consume it can affect just *how* we live in
many major ways. Reciting mindful eating improves digestion,
helps eliminate junk foods, curbs overeating and contributes
to more fastidiousness in ones life. This in return helps you
become aware of your intake, feelings, triggers and urges. In
the end, you tend to improve your mental outlook just as much
as your waistline. As you experience the awareness attained
from mindful eating you may find the desire to improve spreads
way into the corners of your existence.

3

Chapter Three

Preparing For Mindful Eating

Mindful eating is not an event but a journey, a ritual you can carry wherever life takes you. I must warn you that mindful eating is in now way a quick fix to a given problem. It is a commitment, and like anything worth having, it takes faithful regular engagement to achieve deep-seated results. To encounter success make it part of your everyday life. It's immensely helpful to prepare well in anticipation of the practice.

One of the most important keys to the success of the mindful eating journey is preparation. Before you jump in, make sure that you have prepared well reap the benefits right from the start. Many people see others practicing mindful eating and dive in without proper preparation, then after a few weeks or even days, they are back where they began, chomping away without a clue and mostly likely negatively opinionated to the ritual as a result. If you want to enjoy the journey longer than the urge to regress, then get prepared to get prepared before you start. Here are a number of things to help you lay the groundwork:

Know Your Why

Why do you want to practice mindful eating in the first place? This is the most important question to ask yourself before you start practicing anything new. It will help you lay clear plans for all the other aspects of your new habit. Many people start considering diets, extreme exercise and other fads when they encounter a number of problems such as excess weight, struggling with eating, mental strife or feeling out of shape. All these are important reasons to adopt a sensible new health plan, but they often are not enough of an anchor to sustain any newly acquired practice.

Mindful eating is a perennial practice. It is not a hasty remedy for deep seated problems. Keeping this in mind along with your reason why, will help you tie the ritual to a more meaningful, and therefore deep rooted goal. For example, if you feel that practicing mindful eating will help you lose weight, you need to ask yourself; why you want to lose weight? **Hint:** *There more to it than fitting in skinny jeans or rocking your old High School T-Shirt at the reunion.* Who else will be affected by your choice either way? and what next? What happens when the weight is achieved? Then what? Trust me, doing so will really help you get crystal clear on your 'why'.

Plan What to Eat

Depending on your "why", the next step to take is to plan what to eat. Mindful eating doesn't require that you flip up your diet and throw out all the things you love right from day one. However, a dietary overhaul will come instinctively as time goes on. With that being said, making a plan and deliberately choosing your dishes for the day will help you achieve your goals. Remember: Meal prepping sets up up for success but don't let a lack of planning stop you for now. If you are feeling overwhelmed start where you are! Refinement will come in time.

A great place to start if you cook at home is meal planning at least 2-3 evening meals for the week and doubling them. Giving you enough left overs for lunch. Even more refinement, start every meal with two cups of greens as the base. There's no simpler way to polish up your diet than that.

Similarly, if you eat out most of the time you should consider planning. This is because it's preferable to know what you will have for breakfast, lunch, and dinner before you leave your house. That way you won't be inclined to feel hunger and grab the first thing you see. Remember, the food you eat makes you - literally. *How* you eat your food has a huge impact on the digestion and your mental state but ultimately it is the actually choice and range of food you eat that will offer up the nutrients that shape your body. For this reason, it's a good idea to seek out restaurants near work that meet the needs of your new practice of intuitive eating, those with a wider range of fresh options, or at the very least, a salad selection. You may even need to ditch your favorite restaurant if it doesn't serve you in your new practice. Be prepared: mindful eating will eventually magnify flavours! Knowing where you will eat is as important as knowing what you will eat if you eat out for most meals. Therefore, prepare for anything and make plans early so that you are in the know when it comes to those places that will support your new ritual.

Know When to Tend Eat

Mindful eating deals with self-awareness. Therefore, before you dive in, give some time to a little self-analysis to better understand your current eating habits. When do you usually have your meals? What motivates you to eat? What do you love eating? (be honest!). Who do you eat with? How do you feel when you eat? Where are you when you eat? Answering these questions will help you plan when to eat.

By now it's clear what with this practice comes a change to your eating habits. This can be a real struggle without planning, but it doesn't have to be. Following these preparatory tips will ease you into your new and improved way of eating and planning will become an elementary part of it as time goes on. With this in mind, lets find out when you usually eat. Do you eat three times a day or do you eat anytime you have food? Do you eat when you are hungry or do you only have time in the day to eat 1 or 2 larger meals?

Next, you need to find out the *type* of foods you tend to reach for. This alone could give you an idea of how to achieve your goal but most importantly is connected to the time and frequency with which you eat. People who eat snacks and light meals tend to eat more frequently than those who prefer large heavy meals. And finally, give thought to why you eat the foods that you do. This will help you understand your given frequency of eating at present. People who eat only when they are hungry tend to eat fewer meals per day than those who eat for emotional reasons or by blindly following an often unavoidable set timetable due to work and school scheduling.

During this stage gather as much information about your eating habits as you can think of then use the information to prepare a tailored eating plan for yourself. Include both main meal times and snack times. This plan will help you avoid emotional eating and be more focused on your hunger rather than the schedule. This is a key factor in reducing over-consuming and mastering mindful eating.

Plan When You Will Eat

Thoroughly ruminating on food while perceiving and tasting the entire spectrum of flavors, instinctively leads to leisurely dining over a more extended duration than you would otherwise do. With that in mind, it's astute to allow for sufficient time when mindfully eating. Wolfing down lunch in 5 minutes won't work here. You need more time even for a tea break or an evening snack. Therefore, advance mealtime scheduling can be very helpful. Just think, with all this active meditation woven into the tapestry of your day, you are going to be reducing stress and gaining clarity at multiple points in your routine lineup. You'll be a bona-fide mindful eating guru in no time!

If you leave the house for the day, then it's a smart choice to organize your grub so it can seamlessly blend into your schedule. Taking a work lunch with your colleagues can eat into your agenda if your regular place is located several miles away. Opting for an alternative a little closer to your workplace or packing a lunch might be a more suitable option as you refine your intuitive eating. It may seem like a social challenge at first, but remember your 'why' and acknowledge just how important this shift in your mindset is for your long-term physical and mental well being. You may even inspire an office wide adoption of the skill which would be a great advantage for everyone on your team and lead to less afternoon 'slumps' for you and your colleagues! If you come across people that try to discourage you from the practice, and you will, again remember your 'why'. Most people have a fear of that which they don't understand and even more anxiety at the thought of standing out from the crowd. Talking to them about your goals and remaining resilient in your pursuit may make you a little bit of a non-conformist for a while. Historically, nothing great ever occurred to those who chose to remain the same as everyone else - stick with it, Pioneer! If your efforts to create consensuses with your lunch-mates hits a wall, make plans to eat elsewhere where you can practice in peace and focus on your goals, not potentially negative conversation. Planning how you will eat is thus an important step to integrate overtime.

Plan Where you Will Eat

To allow for laser focus on the practice, plan to eat with minimum distractions. If you live alone, work from home, take meals mostly at home and barely ever see anyone....then you won't find this to be an issue at all! But, for most of us, friends pop-in from time-to-time, there are children, family members, roomies, workmates and anyone else you interact with that may hold some weight in the decisions regarding meals. If you work long hours outside of your home or on the road, then you may find it almost impossible to eat at home. In such cases, proper preparation and determination will optimize your success and discourage you from scarfing a limp, gas station sammie over your keyboard.

As you plan your day, make note of your days events and if such will require you to eat out or in. The secret to mindful eating is enjoying your food and doing so in relative serenity, therefore aiming for a quality meal enhances the experience and can steer you away from potentially finding yourself with limited options leading to more stress, less pleasure and prematurely swallowing un-chewed bites purely to satiate hunger. If you eat out seek out places that have healthy, fresh options and if you prepare meals at home it's rational that you would work to elevate your cooking skills to further enjoy well balanced and loving prepared meals every time you eat.

<u>Plan How Much To Eat</u>

For most people eating is simple: eat until the food served on your plate is gone. In fact, many of us grew up believing we have to 'clean the plate' in order to leave the table. Well, (Mom), turns out this is a very problematic habit to get into! For many others, eating enough means you are experiencing a full stomach. This also is an less than ideal way to view food and the consumption of food. Mindful eating leads to portion control. You can start that aspect whenever you are ready. Which you will find is quite soon into your practice as you analyze your eating and determine the portion of foods needed to quench your hunger. Soon enough you will serve just the right amount to be satisfied and no more.

Limiting the size of your plate or bowl can really help here. Some people even choose to eat only with chopsticks! It's up to you. The aim of the game here is to strike a balance between adequate nourishment and consuming for the sake of it.

<u>A tip for successful snacking</u>: avoid eating from the package. Instead serve the snack on a plate or bowl that is small enough to eat in one sitting and no more. Think the largest bowl of the house filled with popcorn.. chances are you'll eat the whole thing. A smaller bowl, plus awareness as you consume will avoid this.

Again it's important to note that you can practice mindful eating without at a plan at all, without a change to your current food or meal times and without altering the frequency with which you cook at home or eat out. As you become more accustomed to the ritual, the enhanced tastes and textures of your foods and heeding the signals of fullness, you will naturally shape your diet around that which suits you best and be well prepared from the lessons in this book to do so like a boss!

4

Chapter Four

Putting Mindful Eating into Practice

If you are new to mindful eating then you are probably wondering where to begin. The simplest way to commence is to start at your next meal by slowly eating your food in a way that allows you to enjoy every bite. Just this one step alone will give your body time to take in the most nutrients as you begin the development of a strong relationship with your food. To do this right away, be aware of every moment during your eating. Once you've had a couple of meals this way you can effectively begin to include a number of important steps to enhance your journey.

Get Rid of All the Distractions

If you are eating at home make sure that you switch off the TV. Eating in front of the TV is a sure way to mindlessly eat. Put away all books, magazines, your smartphone and any other possible source of distraction before you serve your food. This is important to ensure that you are not distracted during eating. Mindful eating requires that you focus on your food 100%. Check around the room for anything that may steal your focus from food and get rid of it. This will give you the peace you need to wholly focus on your food.

Be Thankful

The next important step to take is to honor your food, your body and your environment. Once you and your meal are at the table, sit down in a comfortable chair, take in a few deep breaths and say a few words of thanks. It doesn't have to be well prepared or lengthy, just sincere. ***You don't have to follow a particular religion to embrace gratitude.*** Being thankful will enlighten you to your eating patterns and gives you the grace to begin accepting the emotions that you may experience. Reflect on the blessings you have beyond food, good health, your life, and your family among others. During this short thanksgiving session, it will be a great idea to call out every food item you have on your table by name as you give it individual thanks. Calling out the dishes you have by their names will help you get deeply in touch with the food you are going to eat and prepares your body for the tastes and flavors those foods have. This also primes your mind to accept the food before you as delicious and nutritious and one that will provide for all your needs.

Serve Your Food in Modest Portions

Now, if you are eating alone resist the temptation to eat from the first plate you find or, we've all done it, straight from the pan it was cooked in. Instead, take a clean small plate and serve a modest portion for yourself. Smaller portions removes the temptation that may come with staring at a mountain of goodies waiting to be devoured. Instead, you have a reasonable allotment that you can always add to if you still hungry. A large plate with a large pile of food is a recipe for distraction and overeating.

In addition, serving small portions is a great way to avoid wasting food, giving you more left over in your grocery budget for higher quality ingredients.

Eat your Food in Small Bites

Let's eat! Consciously choose to take small bites and drag out each chew. Small bites have big advantages. First, you leave enough room in your mouth for food to thoroughly roll around, mixing with the enzymes in your saliva and contributing to the softening of each morsel for easy swallowing. Your mouth gets way too filled up when bites are too large, sometimes to the extent that you can barely chew. This forces you to swallow food you have not chewed well and prevents your saliva from completing it's step effectively. This negatively affects your digestion as the food you send to the stomach is not yet ready to be processed. In return, the food passes through your digestive system without being properly macerated which ends up limiting the number of nutrients that your body can absorb. Taking small bites helps eliminate this problem so that you can get maximum nutrients and prevent the stomach nasties!

Chew Slowly and Thoroughly

The very essence of mindful eating is in the drawn out chew. This allows you more time to focus on your food so that you can feel the texture, taste, and flavors. Make an effort not to swallow your food until you feel that it has been thoroughly chewed. By this think liquid. This may be difficult at first because perhaps you are used to chewing your food fast and for a short period before swallowing. But with practice, you should be able to master the art. To help you slow down you should consider putting down your spoon or fork in between bites then pick it up to take the next bite and even consider counting a minimum of 20 rotations of the mouth before swallowing. Your bite will be well and truly mush by then!

Engage All Of Your Senses

Bring all your six senses to the table with you when you dine. See and internalize the colors of your food, notice the smell and texture of the food as you take it into your mouth. As you chew feel the differing taste, texture and the sound with every chew. This will make you appreciate the food you are having and remain focused on the food. You may experience interesting emotions, try to allow them to pass without judgement and keep your mind on the bites you are enjoying. Deeper, more conscious breathing while eating will help reduce any arising stress, further engage your pleasure senses and encourage you to take your time.

Constantly Check on Your Hunger Levels

When you deliberately eat at a decelerated pace, you are likely to get earlier signals from your body that you are now full. This is the time to stop eating. This will allow room in your stomach for digestion. Most of the time we eat mindlessly, our thoughts engaged elsewhere as we rely on the brain to go through the motions of a habit we know all too well. This literally distracts your mind from realizing when you are full. In the end, you could end up with a stomach so full that there is no space left for breathing and proper digestion to take occur and we all know how uncomfortable that can feel. Pausing between bites, smaller bites, smaller portions and more deliberate cognizance of the flow of each bite will teach you, rather quickly, when you are satiated without have to bust a button!

5

Chapter Five

Tips for Mindful Eating

Starting and sustaining a life-long mindful eating practice can appear, for many, to be a tall order at first. Especially in the fast paced times of consumption and excess we experience in modern society. In the world today we navigate so many challenges with our various work, school and leisure-time activities, that there is a general complaint of an inability to get a grip on the day-to-day playbook of their regular commitments, let alone eating. Sound familiar? If have difficulty finding time to eat anyway due to an over-stretched schedule, you may find yourself wanting to give up with mindful eating. If you are limited to your food choices as you are not the primary cook in the home, or perhaps you are bound by a certain menu due to allergies, financial or religious constraints, don't worry! You can pick up where you left off at anytime and recommence the benefits without any loss. Maybe you *are* the primary cook in the home and your dining companions are all children, you may spend most of your time taking care of your family and *their* balanced nutrition only to relegate your *own* diet to left-overs and snacks. Relax! Just take it easy on yourself and stay focused on slowly grasping the reigns of your schedule and your food intake wherever you can, because one day, with committed forward momentum, you will. You may have to work toward changing your circumstances to support your mindful eating journey and beautifully, the journey itself will evoke positive change. If you are concerned as to how you will make this whole thing happen.. fear not! Here are a number of important tips to ease you on your way:

Set Realistic Goals

As mentioned earlier in this book, mindful eating is not a rapid solution for any health-related problem. When someone impulsively begins something new only to surrender just as suddenly, the objective is typically short-sighted. A desire for a 'quick fix'. When results fail to manifest in volume after a week or so a new approach is adopted and the old one is abandoned. Usually, in these cases, there's additional struggles going on like weight problems, fuzzy goals, self-worth or confidence issues, or even common stress and anxiety. Therefore an urgency is applied to hastening the results of mindful eating. As you can imagine, this doesn't work. Mindful eating works it's magic on it's own terms and is a long life journey that requires developing discipline and commitment for you to reap its spectrum of benefits. For this reason, you need to set realistic goals. For example, if you are overweight and you want to use mindful eating to attain a healthy body then a more practical range of goals could be keeping up with your kids, sitting comfortably on a plane, crossing your legs easily, tying your shoes without distress, feeling at ease on the beach, enjoying meals without subsequent bloat and discomfort. This realistic approach is considerably more practical than "to lose 50lbs in two weeks" which is frankly enough to scare anyone into a bag of donuts. Start by tying your practice to commonsense goals and you will be able to extend the duration of your new custom long into the future, eventually with minimal effort.

<u>Start Small</u>

Mindful eating comes with an adjustment to your eating habits. As you may have experienced yourself, permanent modification of habit in your life does not happen in a flash, New Years resolutions are a perfect example of this. It takes time and effort on your part to actualize. For this reason, it is important you start small. For example, you may begin by practicing mindful eating with the main meals of the day only, let's say lunch, breakfast and dinner and not any snacks in between. Maybe even just one meal a day if this is within your current bandwidth. This can be very helpful for individuals that work away from home and have a number of snacks with coworkers who are not practicing mindful eating or perhaps time constraints enable only occasion for only quick bites. Alternatively, you may choose to begin your practice of mindful eating at home for the first few weeks to hone the steps and forge a lasting habit *before* transition to meals eaten out. These achievable, micro-steps will give you a strong sense of accomplishment and support you in creating a sustained discipline that will go a long way in improve your life.

Seek Support

A lot of people who start mindful eating end up forgetting all about it in the first few months because of lack of support. If you want to succeed with mindful eating it may benefit you to assemble a network of advocates. In fact, science proves that any new undertaking has double the chance of success when you include an accountability factor. You could request a family member, a colleague, or a close friend so that you can start the journey together giving each other the much-needed support. Perhaps even reaching out to a successful mindful eater and asking them to mentor you, and talk you through the more challenging patches. There are also a number of groups on social media dedicated to mindful eating. You could join one that best suits you and share your experience with others on the same journey. This way you will remain motivated even if at times you may be forced by circumstances in your life not to eat mindfully a meal or two in a week.

Make your Food Choices Carefully

One key to success with mindful eating is choosing the food that you love. If you are having something you prefer then you will find it easy to chew it for longer luxuriating in every bite. However, if you are eating something you dislike then you will struggle to chew slowly and may end up just swallowing the food as quickly as possible to be done with it. You may also discover that 'sloth-like' handling of fast-food you may have *once* enjoyed, *now* leaves a less than desirable flavor when the customary 5-chew-swallow turns into the 20-chew-swallow of mindful eating. Quality food becomes a much higher priority when cuisine is going to be hanging around your taste buds for much that longer. If you cook at home make sure that you shop for the best ingredients you can afford. If you eat out make sure that eat at restaurants that underpin your resolution and always order something you will relish in.

Identify and be on the Lookout for your Eating Triggers

The ideal aim of mindful eating is to eat enough of the most nutrient dense foods, when we are hungry and to engage in the process in a fully present manner. However, many people eat for a wide variety of reasons that include none of these. If this is you, then it's probably time to put your food triggers under the microscope and reconnect you to the right track. For example, if stress pushes you to eat then you won't eat mindfully because you are too focused on what is stressing you to even notice how you are eating. Try learning to **cope** with emotional triggers in other ways such as: some kind of exercise, pushups, walking, jogging, weights, or yoga. Perhaps a podcast, motivational speech, calling a friend or playing with your pet. EMotional eating goes deeper than self-discipline and is often rooted in conditioning, which can make breaking the habit extremely challenging. Doing something different, trying some of the ways suggested and adding more to your list, can help you learn to choose food for the right reasons and elevate your serenity at the same time.

Create a Healthy Eating Environment

Many of us struggle with eating habits that no longer serve us because whenever we feel hungry we wander through cabinets and shovel in the first thing we find in random places around the kitchen. Also, with a plethora of home delivery services, we can practically eat anything, at anytime, whether we truly need it or not. Now that we have planned our meals, organized our day, evaluated our support system and leveled up the 'fixings', it's time to look around at the places where we dine. We've cleared the dining room or counter and limited distractions, here is where we cast our attention to the surfaces on which we eat. Lap eating is fine, but dining at a table or counter is better as you can typically put down your fork without concern of upsetting the precarious balance of the tray on your thighs..In addition, it's ideal to create a comfortable space, soft lighting, music, cushy chairs. Why not? We don't have to save the best china for once a year! You can enjoy every meal as if it's Thanksgiving. This will create an ambiance conducive to consciousness, plus you'll feel like royalty during this special time carved out of your day just for you. Eating out? Identify restaurants with cozy, or at least, tranquil settings. Bright lights, austere plastic tables and hard molded booths are designed to be functional, and by fast-food design, just uncomfortable enough that you'll scoff quickly and get your bum out of them ASAP.

Indulging once in a while is not a Big Deal

"That's it! No more variety or fun foods for you!" Kidding! You aren't relegated to kale and quinoa from this day forward, unless you love it of course but recognize that consistency with mindful eating will indeed bring about improved results. However, go ahead and indulge once in a while. Forbidding anything in life creates a stronger desire than ever before. Have you ever noticed that? Relish every mouthful and take pleasure in the moment. Once in a while you may find yourself having to gobble up food at work or a party, at the airport or between meetings. It is not a big deal to go off the rails once in a while. All you have to do is remember to come back and continue with the journey.

There are so many experts and information regarding mindful eating. Don't be pushed in a corner by believing you must follow all the rules out there. Remember, you are seeking to establish a deeper relationship with yourself through meals. Make sure that you use common sense to determine what is best for you.

6

Chapter Six

The Benefits of Eating With Family and Friends

Eating with others, especially close family and friends, has a profound impact that ultimately leaves an impression on your biological, psychological and social well being. When you break bread with others you are able to connect in a memorable way that can fill your heart and your belly have a palpable influence on your tranquility. Likewise, eating in the company of others can support new habits, as you strive to find common ground with your table-mates through the contentment of meals. Capitalizing on these aspects can further your new skills. Here are some of the ways eating with family and friends can help you improve your mindful eating:

Bring your Mind to the Dining Table

Eating with others satisfies a basic human need for social

interaction. When there are others to talk to and share jokes with as you eat, you are more likely to be aware of your surroundings than when you dine alone. The truth of the matter is eating alone can go both ways; offering up the solace required for pure focus or the silence that can give way to thoughts of loneliness or even alienation. Not always, but companions generally bring about a release of tension and act almost as a 'glue' after a rough day or during a stressful season in ones life.

Filter Common Distractions

Eating alone lends itself to the convenience of grabbing a stool at the counter while perhaps even multi-tasking or getting up periodically to perform household chores. You may be inclined to eat by your computer as you scroll through, and even complete, projects, work or emails. Perhaps you are a familiar sight on the couch, watching television and robotically spooning in food at meal times. Such deviations make it impossible to practice mindful eating. When you eat with others you are likely to set the table well, mute or turn off the TV, shut down your computer and put off doing household chores that would otherwise detract from the gathering and enjoyment of the meal.

Gratitude as a Group

One of the most important elements of mindful eating is being thankful for what you have. We tend to be more inclined to give gratitude for meals when others are present. Although many people are lost in the worries of this world, often when you eat in a group there's a likelihood that thanks for both the meal and the company will arise in some capacity or another. It is common for families, groups and even close friends to say a prayer or to speak their gratitude before a meal. Thanking the cook is a typical way to start a meal and always appreciated. If this has not been a practice of up to this point, now might be a good time to begin the tradition.

Curbing the Cram

Eating with others has a way of decompressing those present which goes a long way in aiding your mindful eating practice. When you eat with others you are more likely to engage in beautiful conversation about important issues that you face, catch up with one another and even share jokes. All these small talks between bites work magic in curbing the tempo of eating, reducing the chance of cramming bites. This is an especially helpful example for children who will benefit tremendously from the automaticity of mindful eating starting so young in life and could even prevent choking as they see adults taking smaller bites and more care with food. Furthermore, *you* too will generally chew your food more thoroughly when in company. This is because as you follow the conversation and it's highlights and pauses, you will hold your food in the mouth much longer before swallowing. Have you ever noticed this when someone is telling a good story over dinner? As we've discussed, this goes a long way in aiding your digestion. In addition, you may also take the opportunity of participating in the conversation to practice putting down your folk or spoon in between bites, consciously relaxing and breathing in the moment.

<u>Respite as you Bite</u>

As mentioned, solo dining can lead to either **more** <u>or</u> **less** focused eating. This is especially the case at the onset of your mindful eating pilgrimage. The truth is that mastering mindful eating is not an easy task. In most cases, when you start mindful eating you have no idea what it even means to eat slowly and chew your food more thoroughly. Most likely you have never tried breathing with ease and relaxing as you eat. When you eat with others in a comfortable setting with no time constraints, you relax and breathe easy in between bites as typically there are few distractions.

The Challenges of Eating with Others

As with most beneficial things, there are some challenges to consider! Mindful eating requires a lot of concentration from you and therefore it is important to take note of any hinderances that may prevent you from mastering the practice. Some of the major challenges of eating with others include the following:

Distraction

The television or radio are obvious sources of distraction. However, the truth is that when you eat with others, they too can be a major source of distraction! If you have a family member or friend that talks loudly or dominates the conversation, you may find yourself captured more by the content of the dialogue that the cadence of reciprocal conversation. An emotive topic may bubble to the surface that might irk you enough to unsettle you and put a 'fang' where your 'fork' should be... It is thus important to be on the lookout for conversations that could steal your focus and, if possible, know the guest list in advance. This way you will be prepared to remain focused even when 'Aunt Shirley' do her best to distract you.

Setting the Pace

So...how to eat slowly when others may be setting the pace of consumption? Imagine you are running late to have a quick bite before heading back to work. Your colleagues take the lead and order something that is easy to eat. They then proceed to blitz their burger so that they are done in a matter of minutes. What will you do? Will you hold your ground and let them head back to work as you proceed with your mindful eating? The answer for many people here is no. Why? Well, of course, you may need to be back at a certain time but generally we tend to be influenced by others in many ways than we wittingly acknowledge or admit. For this reason, chances are you will overlook your desire to practice mindful eating and go-with-the-flow and pace of the group. If you think you might have a tendency to conform to the affable masses then perhaps head back to the earlier sections of the book and reconsider where and with whom you eat.

Discouragement

In many cases others take note when you start something new. Not everyone is ready when you 'shake up the glitter' in the snow globe of your normal life! Fortunately, those that know you well will most likely understand and in many cases, offer up genuine support. However, you may come across well meaning friends, family and colleagues who will appear to try everything they can to discourage you. Bias opinions usually come from one of three places: ignorance, failure or fear. It is in our nature to either *encourage* or *discourage* others. Therefore don't be surprised if there are a few in your network that try to dissuade you from this new practice. Creating a new normal isn't for everyone. Go ahead and meditate while you chew alarmingly slowly, Ninja of the Nibble!

Ceding Control

When eating together with others you may be forced to cede control of the contents of your plate. A perfect example of this is eating with family where you are not the chef. This may also be the case when you eat out, when invited to family gatherings or when your spouse or partner takes charge of preparing meals. The good news is that by talking to others and letting them know of your mindful eating journey you will give yourself a little bandwidth to take charge of your own pace at the very least. Over time, you may consider cooking or offering up preparation of a side dish, or course. As you develop your commitment to the practice you may find that both yourself and those you dine with begin to take your new manner of eating into consideration at meal times.

Quick Tips When Eating with Others

Ground Yourself – Start by taking a few deep breaths and give thanks. Take notice of your food, the room and everyone in it. If the conversation changes come back to this method of grounding and begin again

Set the Pace – When you eat at a slower pace others are likely to take a cue and adopt your pace. Try not to let your meal-mates take the lead.

Order First – Be ready to order first. As mindful eating includes food choices, choose the healthy foods that you like and supports your practice. Doing so sets the tone of food to be ordered on the entire table and influences the choices of those that order after you. Letting others go first will mean that you are likely to be influenced to order foods that may not be healthy or you may not like.

Chose Something Familiar – Eating with others can be a brilliant opportunity to try new food, new flavors and just about any new thing on the menu. The problem with this is that if you are just beginning your mindful eating journey this can set you back if it turns out to be a dish you dislike. Wait until you've been down the path of mindful eating before you check out something new and obscure on the menu.

Actively Participate in the Conversation – When you eat with others there can be multiple conversations occurring at the same time. Remember to breathe, put down your fork between bites and actively listen as you chew, using short chewing breaks to actively participate and take pleasure in your experience.

Whenever Possible Chose your Company Wisely – Conversation can be a strong determinate of your emotional state during meals. While you are in the early stages of your practice it can behoove you to dine with those that support rather than discourage you. Of course, this may not always be possible but if the guest list is in your control...you may want to exert it.

7

Chapter Seven

Commonly Asked Questions

Q - I am already too thin, now if I practice mindful eating, what will happen to my weight?

A - Mindful eating is not a weight loss or weight gain process. With the consideration that goes into every meal using this method, you will learn to naturally find the weight that is right for you. Less time focusing on your weight and more presence with the balance of nutrients and emotions surrounding meals, will help you establish an healthier relationship with food and an equilibrium in your body.

Q - Is mindful eating a diet?

A - No! No fads, no quick fixes, no restrictions. Mindful eating aims to undo the 'all-or-nothing' approach many of us have adopted over the years. It has no strict rules on what to eat and when to eat what. Instead, you make your own choices and savor eat bite without guilt, shame or a negative inner commentary . The only rules are to be present, eat slowly, chew until the mouthful is liquid before swallowing and to consume each meal without judgement.

Q - How does awareness help other areas of my life?

A - By bringing mindfulness to the table we are teaching ourselves to be less driven to by emotional decision making. Many of us were taught to either punish or reward ourselves with food, instilling a host of emotions both positive and negative around food. Learning to approach your nutritional intake in a stoic and observant manner will lead to a similar application in other areas of your life. Ultimately, supporting calmer more thoughtful approaches to otherwise emotive circumstances.

Q - How can mindful eating help my food addictions?

A - We tend to reach for foods that are high in sugar, salt and fat when we are emotionally driven to eat. Science proves that when we attempt to restrict intake those desire become even more explicit. The beginning step of mindful eating is to analyze your eating habits and the forces behind such habits. Identifying that which triggers the urge and observing your intake as a result, can help you plan alternative stress-reduction measures and meals but also give solid reason to the food selections you are making. Couple this with the non-restrictive menu of the mindful eater, and you have choice without the accompanying guilt or shame, giving you concrete support in breaking the chain of compulsive eating.

Q - Mindful eating has no rules about the foods I should eat. Does it mean I can now eat anything I want?

A - Yes!. With mindful eating, you can eat anything you want. In fact, it is proven that strict rules are unsustainable for long-term wholesome eating. For this reason, the very act of ***slowing down to fully observe your presence of mind with every bite*** will, with time, instinctively lead you to more nutritious and balanced choices. Indulging in things from time to time is up to you. Just ensure you apply the same calm, present, slow composure!

Q - Do I have to be a practicing Buddhist or Hindu to practice mindful eating?

A - Not at all. Mindful eating has roots in the spiritual world but is a choice anyone can adopt. It has been proven to scientifically aid any human body and that includes all of us.

www.ingramcontent.com/pod-product-compliance
Lightning Source LLC
Chambersburg PA
CBHW051125250726
48655CB00007B/2899